The ½ Plan

This is NOT a Diet Fad,
It is a Lifestyle Change

The ½ Plan

This is NOT a Diet Fad,
It is a Lifestyle Change

Chrystyne Tran, MSPA-C

To order additional copies of this book, contact:
Xlibris Corporation
1-888-795-4274
www.Xlibris.com
Orders@Xlibris.com
95296

CONTENTS

Living a healthier lifestyle at a healthier weight for a lifetime . . .

As a physician assistant, I take care of patients and their medical needs on a daily basis. Day in and day out, I see how diabetes, high blood pressure, and high cholesterol can rob a person's health, leading to heart attacks, strokes, peripheral artery disease, kidney failure, etc. Of course, in some cases, these conditions are genetic, but unfortunately, in our American society now, majority of the cause of these conditions is due to being overweight or obese.

When I first diagnose a patient with diabetes or hypertension, counseling about eating a healthier diet and exercising more is always important. Usually, if their condition is not life-threatening at the time, we would discuss how to incorporate healthier food choices, portion control, and daily exercise into their routine. Also, I would mention that if they don't make the changes, then the only option is to give them medications. They would then swear that they WILL lose weight because they don't want to take medications. Patients then leave the office feeling very motivated to make "the change" and I feel encouraged for them. Unfortunately, at follow up visits, the percentage of those who did make real changes in their lifestyle to lose the weight is very low and majority of these patients eventually have to take medications for their conditions. It is very discouraging and defeating as a healthcare provider to write a prescription for a reversible condition.

Also, I have patients who come in asking for the "magic" pills to lose weight. As you know, there is no such thing. There may be diet pills available on the market, but the effectiveness of these pills are temporary, meaning as long as you take them, you lose weight. And if you stop taking them and continue your unhealthy lifestyle, you will gain the weight back and sometimes more. We all know this yo-yo effect. Also, do you want to be dependent on pills for rest of your life and this is without mentioning the potential side effects of these pills. This also applies to those who seek weight loss surgery without making real changes to their lifestyle. If you are not trained to eat less and exercise more prior to these methods, then you have a very high chance to gain all the weight back.

There are patients who tell me that starving themselves or going vegetarian for a month is the only way they know how to lose weight. You may lose the weight during this time period but similar to the "magic" pills, these changes are unrealistic and unsustainable.

Of course, the majority of Americans who are obese is due to overeating and lack of exercise, but there are some medical diseases that can cause someone to gain weight that is not associated with poor diet. These conditions my include hypothyroidism, Cushing's disease, long term effects of steroid medications, etc., which do need medical intervention. Even if you do have these medical conditions that may slow down your weight loss efforts, it would not hurt to follow this plan to live a healthier life.

Also, there are other obstacles I hear from patients which may be preventing them from effectively losing weight, such as not being able to afford healthier meals. Therefore, they have to eat fast food which is high in carbohydrates, salt, and fat. Consider this, at a fast food restaurant, for a family of 4, it would cost an average of $20/meal compared to a prepared dinner at home with lean meats, veggies, and starch, which can be half the price. In addition, I often hear that patients overeat due to depression or boredom. Definitely, these emotional conditions will affect our habits, but think about this. If you are depressed and bored, what are you accomplishing by overeating? Nothing!!! You will just make yourself more depressed as you gain more weight and you will definitely not cure the boredom issue. If depression is a problem, talk to your doctor and get some help. Also, if you start eating healthier and exercising more, you will feel better about yourself and improve your outlook. If boredom is your problem, then get a hobby. Learn a new activity, like playing tennis, golf, karate or go hiking, swimming, running. Even non-physical activities like knitting or scrapbooking is good because you are actively exercising your mind. For this one, you will only be limited by your imagination.

The third common obstacle I hear from patients is that they don't have time to be healthier/lose weight. I know, as a mom, all our waking hours are devoted to our work and our family. Taking care of yourself is probably the last thing on your mind. Any free time is reserved for much-needed sleep. I completely understand that. However, if you can't reserve that extra ½ hour/day to exercise or commit to making healthier choices for yourself, then what happens when you become diagnosed with diabetes, high blood pressure, high cholesterol and suffer from a stroke or heart attack. At that point, you can no longer take care of your children or family. Working with my senior patients everyday, I realize that the best gift you can EVER give your children and family is for YOU to stay healthy. If you don't, you will then burden them with healthcare costs, time off work to take you to the doctors, or even burying you before seeing your grandchildren. If you don't make the commitment now, when will you?

On the positive side, I have seen patients be successful with losing weight by eating less and exercising more. I think the main difference for those who succeed vs. those who fail is due to several factors. The ones who seem to succeed have made a commitment to themselves to change, even when it gets hard. They realize that their current lifestyle cannot continue. They no longer will accept being overweight or obese as their "normal". They no longer make excuses to why they cannot eat less and move more to lose weight. They understand that weight loss is a lifetime commitment. It is not just a 3-6months process. Just think, it took you maybe 5-10 years or more to have gained all your current weight, so it will take time to lose weight. But with each week, you will see 1-2 pounds weight loss, so you will need to continue day by day to lose that 20-30pounds. Successful weight loss is a lifetime process.

We all know "what to do" to lose weight like eating less and moving more. This plan is a step by step "how to" guide to achieve the goal to live a healthier lifestyle at a healthier weight for a lifetime . . .

CHRYSTYNE TRAN, MSPA-C

The intention of my plan is for everyone.

I equate overeating and inactivity to smoking cigarettes. It is a habit. We have to first recognize the behavior/habit. Secondly, it is up to each individual to decide if it is a habit that they want to change or not. If someone does wants to live healthier but will not put in the time and have the willpower to make the steps to stop smoking, then nothing can be done. It is up to each individual to decide and commit themselves to this plan or not. Everyone will quit smoking on their own terms, so will losing weight. It is the individual's CHOICE to change or not. As an adult, if your cause of obesity is not a medical condition, then it is your CHOICE to remain overweight/obese. Even though you have "done every diet plan out there" and "really don't eat a lot" and still haven't lost weight, it is because you are not making the right change.

For example, as in school, if you want to get good grades, you have to commit to studying. You can say you did sit at your desk for 1-2 extra hours to study for the test, but if you still had the TV on and texting your friends at the same time, then that extra 1-2 hour effort doesn't equate to much on the test the next day. But if you were to turn off the TV and phone while studying the next time and focus on good study habits, then the results will definitely be better. Weight loss is the same thing. There is no magic to this. We all expect a miracle from potions and secret tricks to lose weight because we don't want to put in the hard work. We have to get back to the basic habits of good eating and activity. If you have good studying habits in elementary school, then it will benefit you in junior high, high school, college, and life as well. So, if you start changing the basics of your lifestyle to lose weight, then it will help you keep the weight off for the rest of your life.

There is no secret or magic weight loss wand, you just have to want it bad enough. Again, in my practice, I have 2 sets of patients when it comes to weight loss. The ones who are successful are the ones who realize that their diabetes, high blood pressure, cholesterol problem is their own doing and they are willing to make the sacrifices of time and hard work to make the changes. Others give excuses or don't want it bad enough. And that is okay, too. They may not be ready to commit yet, therefore we have medications for those individuals. For those you do the plan and make the changes from Rule 1 to Rule 10 and still have to be on medications, that is okay, too because your heart will appreciate the lesser weight.

Furthermore, another analogy that can apply to weight loss is building pyramids. Everyone wants to get to the top of the pyramid to lose weight but no one wants to help build the pyramids. In order to build the foundation to your own "healthy lifestyle/weight loss" pyramid, you have to build the bricks at the bottom layer first. With each bottom brick, it will be harder to carry because you are not used to it, but as you continue to build your layers, you will be stronger and the same bricks will be easier to carry. If one of your bricks is knocked off by a "life wind/obstacle", at least the bottom layers are intact and you just need to try harder and put that brick back on again. The process is slow and methodical, but it is strong. Everyone will build their pyramid at a different time and each pyramid may be a different color, but we all have the same goal, which is to get to the top.

This plan is not a "diet". The term diet implies that it is a short term process, for example, to be on a diet to lose 10pounds to get into that dress for an upcoming wedding. After the wedding, then you get "off the diet" and gain that 10pounds back and sometimes more. I know, you don't purposely plan to gain that weight back, but somehow it always does. Also usually the term "diet" implies restricting yourself from something, like all sweets, meats, junk food, sodas, etc. Restricting these items from your diet 100% is not realistic. When we restrict ourselves from these items to lose weight, then once we allow ourselves to eat these items again, naturally, you will gain the weight back again. On this plan, you can still enjoy your pizzas, ice cream, steaks, etc., but just eat less of it.

Everyone can lose weight if you really make the efforts, but the hardest part is to keep the weight off. My goal of the plan is for you to establish a healthy lifestyle, so that you will be able to keep your healthy weight a lifetime. Naturally, as we age, we will gain about 3-5 pounds each year without making any changes at all. Blame it on our aging metabolism. The problem with America's obesity problem is a lifestyle of overeating, inactivity and need for instant gratification. I want to slowly give you a step-by-step guide on how to eat less and move more to live a healthier lifestyle at a healthier weight. The process will be slow and gradual, but I ask for your patience. By losing weight slowly, it allows your body to acclimate to the changes better and keep the weight off. You should see changes on a weekly basis. Also, by losing weight by changing your lifestyle, there is a better chance for you to keep the weight off.

This program is different from other programs because there is no calorie counting. There is no crazy 2hour work out sessions at the gym. There is no pain and risk of surgery like weight loss surgery. There is no workout equipment you have to buy. You don't have to drink a pill or crazy concoction of hot sauce and vinegar. Since this plan targets lifestyle and everybody's lifestyle/family is different, each change you implement should just be a modification of your current habits, not a complete change. In other words, you will be able to eat the type of foods you are currently eating and do the activities you normally do, but just modified. I want to go back to the basics with retraining our lifestyle to eat less and move more.

If you eventually decide to do weight loss surgery or take diet pills, you can follow this plan to modify your lifestyle to optimize your success and weight loss.

This plan is also for those who are at their "ideal weight" as well. Even though you are at a good/ideal weight, it does not mean you are practicing healthy habits. For example, a good friend of mine who works a busy schedule, will eat chips and drink soda all day and would eat out majority of her meals at restaurants. Thanks to her amazing metabolism, she is skinny and beautiful, but we are not all blessed like her. With my plan, the goal for someone like her, is not to lose weight, but to make healthier choices. These individuals will feel healthier and have more energy. Also, with the added exercise, they may lose inches around their belly and gain more muscle mass.

This is how the plan works.

Every 2 weeks, you will read a new chapter about a lifestyle challenge to implement in your life. I will also supply you with concrete examples on "how-to" implement the changes. I would like you to monitor your weight on a weekly basis because I want you to be aware of the weight losses and gains as you go through the program. Weigh yourself preferably on Saturday morning, first thing in the morning before breakfast, then write it down on a calendar. Our weight naturally fluctuates throughout the day, so that is one reason I don't want you to weigh yourself more than once a week. Also, don't be discouraged if your weight fluctuates in the first few weeks/months. It is because your body has not adjusted yet. Be patient and stick with the plan. Also remember, the more overweight/ obese you are, then the faster you would lose weight initially, compared to someone who is less overweight. For those who are not overweight, then the purpose of monitoring your weight is to focus on maintaining your weight. During the first two weeks we will implement Rule 1. After the 2 weeks, then you can add Rule 2. Therefore, you will continue Rule 1 and add Rule 2. Each rule will build on another, so we never get rid of any rules as we continue. Some rules will be harder to implement in your life than others, but try your best. If we come across a Rule, like eating 3 smaller meals, which you have already incorporated in your life, then you will not have to do anything new that week, but just continue the Rules you have learned. Once you reach your "happy" weight, you can stop adding new rules. You will just need to continue the lifestyle changes you already made to maintain your "happy" weight.

Because we are all busy with personal and family commitments, I know adding another commitment is a big ordeal. I want to try to make it simple as much as possible for you. This plan is intended for only Monday through Friday. Assuming that you work a Monday thru Friday type of a job, it is already a routine. So, by applying the changes to a routine, it will be easier to implement. On the weekends, our schedule is usually busy and never a routine, so I don't expect you to follow all the rules during Saturdays and Sundays. The only thing I request during the weekend is to continue Rule #1, which is to eat 1/2 what you are already eating at that time. If you wish to do the changes 7days/week, then that is up to you. For those who work irregular schedules, then it will be harder, but still do-able. What you can do is still apply all lifestyle modifications on M-F, "off" on weekends, except for Rule #1.

Before starting the Rules, there are 4 things I would like you to do. First, I would like you to purchase a digital scale. The digital scale will be able to give you an accurate reading each time. Second, find a partner to work with you. Having a partner allows you to be accountable to someone else. We tend to always give ourselves excuses about eating right and exercising, but having a partner in crime allows you to be honest. Also, you can each push and inspire each other. Third, I want you to finish this sentence: I want to be healthier because_____. Please write this sentence on 2 note cards; put one in your wallet to carry with you at all times and the second, stick it on your mirror, so you can remind yourself each day to keep you motivated. Although this step may be silly, it is a necessary step. It will be a constant reminder to continue and keep you motivated. Some examples of motivating factors are: to live longer, to have a baby, to stop some medications . . . . it is up to you.

Fourth, everybody has the goal of losing that 20-30 pounds, but I want you to set your goal to lose 5pounds at a time. It will be more attainable and you feel more accomplished as you make each change. Once you get to your first goal, set another 5pound goal.

CHRYSTYNE TRAN, MSPA-C

This book is not meant for you to read in its entirety at one time. I just want you to read a new rule every 2 weeks. During the 2 weeks, you will try to incorporate the changes in your lifestyle. If you feel you really haven't embraced the rule, then give yourself another 1-2 weeks. It is completely up to you.

It is ironic to think that we are supposed to eat to survive, but now people are dying early because of eating too much. We have to change that.

Lifestyle and Health Assessment

Before you start the changes, I would like you to do the following questionnaire. This will give you an idea about your overall health. Then do the questionnaire at the end of the plan and see how much you have changed or not . . .

1. Do you feel that you are living a healthy lifestyle already?   Yes/No
2. Do you want to live a healthier lifestyle?   Yes/No
3. Do you feel that you overeat?   Yes/No
4. How many sodas/sugary drink/juices do you drink a week?
    0-2   3-5   6-8   8-10   11-15   16-20   more than 20
5. How often do you bring lunch to work? (Assuming a 5day/week work schedule)
    0   1   2   3   4   5
6. Besides walking associated with your daily working schedule, do you do EXTRA work/activities outside of work?   Yes/No
7. Do you eat 3 meals a day?   Yes/No
8. Do you make a habit to add a small amount of protein in your breakfast, such as low-fat cheese, peanut butter, egg, or low fat lunchmeat?   Yes/No
9. How many hours/day do you spend watching TV or playing video games?
    0   1   2   3   4   more than 5
10. Do you eat in the car?   Yes/No
11. Do you have healthy snacks in the car?   Yes/No
12. How many meals do you eat "out" per week?
    0-1   2-3   4-5   6-7   8-9   more than 10

13. When you do eat "out", do you pay attention to
the type of food or amount of food that you eat?   Yes/No
14. How often do you and your family eat dinner together per week?
    0   1   2   3   4   more than 5
15. How often do you cook/prepare dinner for the family per week that does not require the microwave to cook?
    0   1   2   3   4   more than 5
16. Do you make an effort to have high fiber and
vegetables at each meal?   Yes/No
17. Do you often eat sugary dessert with each meal?
    No   less than ½ of meals   More than ½ of meals   Always
18. Have you been already diagnosed with diabetes, high blood pressure or high cholesterol?
                    Which condition: _____
19. Have you had a physical with your doctor this year yet?   Yes/No
20. Are you ready to make lifestyle changes, lose weight,
and maintain a healthier weight for a lifetime?   Yes/No

If you answer No to #20, then this is not the plan for you

Rule 1

Rule 1 will directly address the problem with overeating. As Americans, we are so fortunate to live in a society where everything is so plentiful, especially food, so we tend to overeat without thinking twice. We think that since the food is there, we should eat it. Also, we are the only society that label food as a good food or bad food. My philosophy is all food is good, it is just the large portion size that Americans are accustomed to that is bad. Often times, while developing this plan, I am asked, "is this _____ (insert food name) good to eat?" My answer always is, "yes, but in moderation".

For this rule, I would like you to *eat half the amount of food that you are already eating* (mainly simple carbohydrates, beef products, processed/ frozen foods, and fast food/restaurant foods). The purpose of the rule is not to restrict any type of foods you are normally eating, but train you to eat less. Initially, you many feel that you are not full, but eventually your stomach will get used to it and you will get fuller sooner. If you do not feel full after the ½ meal, then eat more veggies or a fruit. If you are diabetic, then obviously, you have to also limit the amount of fruits you eat, but eating a ½ of a banana or ½ of an apple to help you fill up, will not hurt. If you feel you are eating in small portions already in your routine meals, then just think of the rule when you eat that piece of cake or 2 scoops of ice cream. Naturally, if you eat half the amount of food, then you only take in half the calories, hence losing weight.

Here is a reference for other food groups that we will discuss as you go through the plan:

1. Lean proteins: fish, skinless chicken (preferably chicken breast, but legs/thighs are okay, too, since it tends to leaner than beef), lean pork (without obvious fat showing), eggs (preferably egg whites, but eating 1egg with yolk/day is okay)
   - also raw nuts that are not coated with sugar/honey (almonds, walnuts, pecans, peanuts) and beans are good sources of proteins as well

2. Low fat dairy: milk, yogurt, cheese
3. Vegetables (aka veggies)/Fruits
4. Carbohydrates
   - Simple carbs: white bread/rice, pastas, donuts, cookies, candies, anything coated with sugar, potatoes, sodas
     (these are the foods I really want you to focus to cut ½ on)
   - Complex carbs: anything that is made of whole wheat, brans, oatmeal, brown rice

5. Oils: if you must eat something fried, it is better to have it pan-fried (fried with a very little amount of oil), then have anything deep-fried
   - Olive oil or canola oil is better than corn oil

Here are some suggestions:

1. If you usually eat 2 portions of rice or pasta, then cut down to one, then fill up with veggies
2. If you usually eat 1 slice of the bread given to you before each meal, then eat ½ of a slice
3. If you usually order a salad for lunch, then ask for the dressing on the side and only add half of it in your salad
4. If you usually go out for a steak dinner once a week, then change it to every other week
   - then try eating half of the bread or potato side dish or substitute it for a second portion of veggies

5. If you usually eat 2 slices of pizza, then cut to 1 slice of pizza and add salad
6. If you usually get a large meal plate, then order for the regular plate OR if it is a better deal to order the large plate, order it and split it with a coworker or save half for the next meal
7. If you usually supersize a hamburger meal, then order the meal with small fries and small drink
   - I know sometimes it is a better deal to get the supersize meal, but remember, it is making you fat and unhealthy
8. If you usually order a dessert when you go out to dinner, then eat only half and share it
9. Try to avoid buffet-style restaurants because you will feel ripped off if you don't eat at least 2 plates of food
10. Another good suggestion given to me by one of my coworkers is when you are filling up your plate at a party or at home, place each food item, so that they don't touch each other and you can see the plate in between your food
11. If you usually buy 2 bags of chips/cookies for the family to snack on each week, try to buy only 1. If you don't buy it and bring it home, there will be less calories to intake

So, basically, you can still enjoy your everyday foods, but just less. In this plan, there is no such thing as restricting any particular type of foods, like No Sugars . . . No Carbohydrates . . . No Fats . . . at all. By restricting your diet in that manner, it makes you crave for that food more. Therefore, at a weak moment when you get that food again, then you tend to overload yourself and gain all that weight back again. Restricting food is unnatural, unless you have made a decision to cut it out for a lifetime, like vegetarians. Our body needs a balanced diet to function.

The only thing you do not have to cut in half are veggies and lean proteins like fish, skinless chicken, and low fat pork. Of course, anything baked, grilled, pan-fried is better than deep-frying.

CHRYSTYNE TRAN, MSPA-C

During this process, I was asked whether you will need dietary supplements/ vitamins during this time, since you are eating less. A person who eats less does not mean that they are more vitamin deficient than someone who eats more. It really lies in the type of foods that you eat. If your meals consist of lean proteins, veggies, dairy products, carbohydrates, then you should be getting adequate daily amount of vitamins and nutrients. During my years as a medical provider, the only patients I have seen with vitamin deficiencies are those with eating disorders and those with a medical condition which may cause them to be vitamin deficient that is unrelated to their diet alone. But in general, whether you are on this plan or not, it would not hurt to take a daily multivitamin, along with Calcium/Vitamin D. I will leave it up to each individual's choice. Remember, my plan is the bare minimum request. If you do above and beyond, you are definitely welcome to.

Rule 2

Congratulations on completing the first 2 weeks of the plan.

We will start Rule 2 this week: ***Walk/jog about 30 minutes every day, Monday-Friday***. This is EXTRA outside of your daily routine activities. I would like you to walk/jog enough to break a light sweat. You may add hand weights if you want to increase the intensity. This rule is the bare minimum which should be done, so if you can do more before or after work, that is definitely up to you.

For example, at my work now, my nurses and I would take a walk around our building the last 30minutes during our lunchtime. So, maybe you can start a walking group/club at work. Or maybe wake up 30minutes earlier in the morning and go on the treadmill (if you have a treadmill) before work. Or walk after dinner with the family. Or take the stairs at work every day instead of riding the elevators. If you have a treadmill/elliptical machine at home, put it in front of the TV. By the time you finish your favorite show at night, your workout is done. See what works best in your schedule.

Sometimes exercise can be seen as a chore, so see if you can wake up 30minutes earlier each day and exercise before going to work. At least, this one "chore" will be done with for the day and you will feel good about yourself the rest of the day. I know how busy it can be at the end of the day with getting dinner ready and kid's bath/homework time, so it can be tough to squeeze that extra 30minutes to exercise by the end of the day.

For our Metro-train people or those who walk at work regularly (like mail carriers), it is up to you if you can add the extra walk/jog. Preferably, yes; if not daily, then try adding 2-3days/week. Basically, the more you move the better.

Remember to continue Rule 1 as well. Again we will do Rule 2 for another 2 weeks. Remember to weigh yourself every Saturday morning and keep a record of it.

Rule 3

Congratulations for finishing the first month of the plan. I know the weight loss is slow but that is okay. Just hang in there. Again, not only is this plan a weight loss program, it is also to focus on living a healthier life with healthier habits. Remember to weigh yourself each Saturday morning.

As for Rule #3: Make a habit to eat 3 small meals a day. No skipping meals, especially breakfast. At each meal, try to make sure you have *lean protein or low fat dairy.*

As know you, in our busy lifestyles we often tend to skip meals and usually breakfast in the meal we often miss. It is important to eat breakfast each morning because we stimulate our metabolism that way. Usually if you don't eat breakfast, then we tend to either grab an unhealthy snack around 9-10am or eat a larger lunch because we are so hungry at that time. I was so guilty of this myself, so I definitely know this cycle. By eating 3 regular meals, your metabolism is always working, which help promote weight loss. Plus, you don't feel sluggish throughout the day. If you are still hungry between meals, pack yourself some fruits or nuts to munch on, rather than grabbing for the donut or chips.

If you are too busy to eat breakfast at home in the morning as you are trying to shuffle the kids off to school, then just pack yourself some breakfast and eat in the car. Or leave some breakfast items at work, such as whole wheat bread, yogurt, bran cereal, milk, etc. at your work/lunch room and eat it when you get to work.

By making sure you have a protein and/or low fat dairy product at each meal, it will help you keep full for a longer period of time. Also dairy products will also help prevent hunger throughout the day. Your stomach does not have a timer and can't tell the difference between breakfast and dinner foods, so don't worry if you happen to eat dinner foods for breakfast, etc. As long as you are feeding your body, it is happy.

Examples of meal plans:

Breakfast:

1. low fat yogurt, a piece of wheat toast with peanut butter, an apple
2. Hard boiled egg, 1-2 slice of cheese, toast, banana
3. sometimes I even make myself sandwiches or last night's dinner for breakfast
4. Eat 10-15 almonds with any breakfast food and you will feel very full for the morning

Lunch:

1. chicken salad
2. Tuna/turkey sandwich
3. leftovers from last night's dinner (which I usually do)

Dinner: focus on adding lean protein with veggies

This obviously requires more meal planning for the week, but try it. Again, my suggestions are the bare minimum, so be creative and make this plan your own.

If you are already eating 3meals/day, then try making breakfast and lunch your larger meals of the day. Have dinner as the smallest meal of the day. By planning your meals this way, this will allow your body and metabolism to process the food/calories during the day when you are most active. By eating a lighter dinner, it may help reduce or prevent acid reflux and indigestion problems as well. I have had some patients do this simple change and they were able to stop their antacid medications.

CHRYSTYNE TRAN, MSPA-C

Rule 4

The next rule will target our dessert "cravings" after meals. It is sometimes automatic after lunches and dinners that we reach for the ice-cream, brownie, cake, cookie, chocolate etc. to satisfy our "sweet tooth". But I want to you to try something new. For Rule 4, **after each meal, instead of grabbing for the processed sweets, eat a fruit instead.** Fruits after each meal will help with your sweet cravings. If after eating the meal and the fruit and you still have room for that cookie or piece of cake, then go for it. But if you do decide to eat the cookie or cake, then remember to only eat ½.

My personal favorite fruit to snack on are apples. In my opinion, I think apples are one the greatest fruits to help you lose weight and stay healthy. Obviously, it is healthy with tons of nutrients and vitamins. But apples are very "dense" as a fruit compared to oranges, so it can be satisfying and filling. The denseness of the apple is fiber, so it will also help regulate your digestive system. I would usually eat an apple in the car on my way to work with a yogurt and have another one after lunch. Apples seem to always be in season, so it is plentiful with many varieties to choose from and often very inexpensive. I truly believe in the saying "an apple a day keeps the doctor away". If you continue to lose weight, it will keep obesity and medicines away as well.

Continue all the other rules, but if you ever forget the week's Rule, just always try to remember at least Rule 1 at each meal.

Rule 5

I hope you have been able to implement the rules in your life. I know some rules are harder than others to implement, while some rules you are already doing. Again, try to modify each rule to your own lifestyle. As for the next rule, the new lifestyle change is to ***bring and eat your own prepared lunches AT LEAST 2x/week.***

The reason I want to implement this rule is often we get too busy with our lives and we don't take the time to pack our lunches for work. Therefore, by lunch time, if we didn't bring anything, then we naturally have to go out to eat. Eating out, most of the time, includes eating fast food, processed foods, larger portions with higher fat and salt contents. This ultimately translates into higher calorie foods. Our own prepared lunches tend to be healthier and smaller portions. Also, if you continue to do this, you will notice that you are saving at least $10/week, which is $40/month, etc.

Try to pack your lunch the night before, since we tend to be too busy in the morning with ourselves and our children to worry about lunch. For me, I even put it in my lunch bag, so it is ready the next day without any fussing at all.

Here are some suggestions:

1. Pack your dinner leftovers for lunch the next day (this is what I usually do); again focus your meals on lean proteins, 1/2 carbs, veggies and fruit

2. If you have a refrigerator/lunch room at work, leave bread (preferably wheat), cheese and low fat/salt lunch meat at work to make sandwiches for lunches

    -   this would be great for days when you don't have dinner leftovers

3. Take turns preparing lunch with your co-workers. For example, you can be in charge of packing lunches for you and your co-worker on Monday and he/she can take care of the packed lunches for you both for Tuesdays, etc.

    -   obviously, if you have more co-workers, then it may be less work

I'm not a fan of packing processed foods, like a frozen pizza, burrito, pasta meals, etc. to heat up for lunch because they tend to be high in fat/salt/calories. But if that is all you have, then try to limit eating the frozen food to 1-2x/week, instead of everyday or cutting the portion down and bringing an extra order of salad or veggies to eat with the meal.

If you must go out for lunch, then maybe share a meal with a friend or eat half and save it for dinner.

Again this rule is to bring lunch AT LEAST 2x/week, but if you can do it more, then Awesome.

Rule 6

To continue the plan, I would like to implement Rule 6 at this time, which is to *cut down our soda/sugary drinks*. I know people and patients who will drink sodas as their main source of hydration instead of water. They tell me the reason they do that is because they "don't like the taste of water". Well, just think about it, if sodas/sugary drinks are all they consume, then obviously water is bland. In this way, water can be an "acquired taste", so it does take time to get used to it and making the change. My trick for blah-bland water is to drink the water cold. It is always more refreshing, I think.

Sodas/sugary drinks are considered empty calories because we don't get any nutritious value from it. Juices definitely are packed with vitamins and nutrients, however, it is overloaded with sugars as well. As a trick, when drinking juices, try diluting half with water. Don't worry about "diluting" the vitamins and nutrients because if you are already doing the other rules, like eating 3 healthier meals a day with a focus on/veggies/fruits, you should be getting plenty of vitamins/nutrients already. As a reminder, if you feel that you are lacking in vitamins/nutrients, at this stage in our lives, it would not hurt to take a daily multivitamin and Calcium with vitamin D (600mg one tab twice a day). Or, just limit juices to breakfast, instead of drinking it casually or drinking it with every meal. I know of one Endocrinologist (doctor who specializes in Diabetes), who would tell her patients to avoid juices and sodas completely because they are loaded with sugars.

We sometimes have a habit to order sodas with our meals or grab for a soda at home/work without even thinking about it. First thing, I would like to recommend is for you to have **a water bottle at your work desk at ALL TIMES**, instead of any soda/sugary drink. I would **NOT recommend putting a water bottle AND a soda** because of course, you would grab for the soda first before thinking about the water. Also, see if you can leave a water bottle in the car. So, if you are thirsty on your ride home, then you will have the water to drink, instead of stopping over and getting a soda.

Other suggestions:

1. For those who have already done this, then maybe reserve the sodas for "special" occasions, like parties, going out for sit-down restaurant meals, etc.
2. If you order a fast-food meal, then order it with the smaller soda choice or just drink half of it. Or order the meal a-la-carte, for example, ordering the burger and small fries separately and ask for a cup of water with it, instead of Meal #1 and getting the burger/fries/soda together. I know that it is sometimes a better deal to get the Meal#1, instead of ordering it separately, but you also have to consider the empty calories you are taking in just because "it is a good deal". These deals are not worth it for your health.
3. If you normally drink a can of soda/day, then just cut it down to Monday/Wed/Fri or just for the weekends
4. If you can't make the big jump from sodas to water, then switching to diet sodas or ice tea instead of regular sodas is a start. If you can eventually wean down to water, then it would be better
5. If you still think water is bland, then they now do have the "vitamin" or flavored water options, which usually have no or low-sugar
6. Add fruit slices to water, like strawberries, cucumbers, lemon/orange slices to flavor the water

7. As for coffee, limit to 2cups/day because it is not the coffee that is high calorie, but the sugar and cream you put in it to make it extra yummy. Try limiting alcohol beverages to less than 2/day as well to reduce your empty calories.

Basically, try to drink LESS soda/sugary drinks than what you are currently doing.

Rule 7

Rule 7 is to incorporate more fresh fruits and veggies to your diet. The first step is to have *a "fruit bowl" at home filled with fresh fruits* available EVERYDAY. The purpose of this step is to have fruits available at all times, so when you are craving for a snack, you will hopefully grab for the fruit instead of the cookies or bags of chips. One tip I do is put fruits, like oranges, apples, grapes, etc. in a VISIBLE section in the refrigerator because these fruits tend to taste better when cold. This also applies to fresh veggies as snacks, too like celery and carrots. So, next time if you feel like a snack, grab the fruit first, then if you still want that cookie or chips, go for it. But remember to eat only ½ portion of the cookie/chips.

Another tip to add fruits and veggies to your life is when you do your grocery shopping each week, go to the produce section of the store first. Look for the seasonal fresh fruits, like apples, oranges, watermelons, etc. Seasonal fruits tend to be less expensive. Buy at least 3 varieties for the week, so you won't feel "bored" with your fruit choices. *Eat at least 2 fruits a day.* What I do is grab a banana or apple in the morning as I head out to work and eat it in the car. Also, I would pack a fruit for me to eat at lunchtime. Also, I would encourage you to consider a "new"/more exotic fruit once in a while to see if it will be something you may add to your regular fruit shopping routine. Consider fruits like mangoes, kiwi, fresh blueberries/raspberries/blackberries, etc.

After choosing your fruits at the store, then buy your veggies for the week. Again, look for the more seasonal items if you can. When you make your lunches or dinner, try to incorporate *1 extra veggie* in your meal.

For example, add celery or cucumbers to your lunch sandwiches if you normally don't. Or add cut mushrooms, zucchinis, or brown onions to your spaghetti sauce or meatloaf if you normally don't.

Try making fruit and veggie trail mixes. I would put some baby carrots, celery sticks, and some strawberries or grapes in a ziplock bags. Put them in the refrigerator ready to go and snack on during the week. Change the variety of fruits and veggies. You can definitely incorporate these mix bags for your children. Surprise them eat day with a new mix for their lunches or snacks.

All this preparation is time consuming, but definitely worth it. I usually reserve 1 hour on Saturdays and/or Sundays to prepare my veggies and fruits for the week. It is faster if you can encourage your children to help or if your children are old enough, this may be one of their chores/ responsibilities for the week to prepare for the family.

Rule 8

Like Rule 7, Rule 8 will address healthier snacking. Snacking is a normal part of our daily routine. The problem with snacking, like eating, is that we sometimes snack on unhealthy foods or eating too much of it. This rule will help focus you to *snack better by snacking less and healthier.* Hopefully, if you are already doing Rule 3 of eating 3 meals a day, then snacking less will not be that difficult because you will be already full.

Here are some suggestions:

1. Buy fruit yogurt, like Yoplait or Gogurt, then freeze them. They make great healthier treats for the kids compared to regular ice-cream. I call them "ice-cream" yogurt at home and my kids are young, so they don't know the difference. It doesn't even seem that they miss the regular ice cream. With older kids, it will be an adjustment but if frozen yogurt is all you have in the freezer, then that is all they will eat. Kids will get their supply of calcium this way as well. Of course, this doesn't eliminate the occasional ice-cream treats, but not on a regular basis.
2. A friend of mine started snacking on Greek yogurt with honey during her breaks at work, instead of the other munchies
3. Buy baked chips, instead of regular fried chips. This will definitely reduce the amount of calories and fat you intake compared to the regular chips. If you buy the baked chips in the smaller/pre-packaged bags, the portions are about the same as the regular chips, so you

can really have a good snack with it. Of course the taste may not be the same, but I like them. Plus, everything and every change is new at this point, so new food change is an acquired taste, such as your new healthier lifestyle is an acquired habit.

4. Buy pre-portioned 100 calorie snacks instead of the regular size. Or you can buy the regular packages and use a ziplock bag to put them in smaller portions yourself.
5. Consider getting a box of pretzels or wheat crackers to eat with cheese or getting a jar of walnuts or almonds instead of automatically reaching for the cookies or chips to stock up for the week.
6. Fruit snacks are great alternatives to candy for children.

Other healthy snacks are dried fruits, with low fat popcorn, low fat cheese, rice cakes, pretzels, or whole grain crackers.

One of my favorite thing to do is buying raw almonds in bulk and roasting a portion of it in the toaster oven; mix it ½ and ½ with dried cranberries and it is a great crunchy and healthy snack. For our diabetics, add ¾ of almonds and less cranberries.

Of course, we don't want to deprive you or your children of chips, candies, cookies, ice-cream, etc. because that is not realistic, but maybe limit to only eating it on the weekends as a "treat" as in my family. Keep these special snacks out of normal sight of you or the children, so there is not that constant temptation every time you open the pantry for bread. Or again, back to Rule #1, if you or they are going to eat it, then eat ½ the portion.

Those suggestions are for the home, but I would also recommend putting a "snack" bag in the car as well. Often times we pack snacks for our kids when they are in the car, so you don't have to stop off somewhere when they are hungry and cranky. So, I want you to apply the same logic for yourself as well. Basically, for foods that are non-perishable like nuts, pretzels, wheat or rice crackers, raisins, etc., have a few of it in glove compartment, so if you get hungry on your way home from work or if you forgot to eat or

CHRYSTYNE TRAN, MSPA-C

bring breakfast, then you can reach for it during a stop light and munch. That will prevent you from stopping at the next fast food place that you see on your way home for a pre-dinner snack. I've been in this trap many times, so I know how that process works. For other snacks like fruits, hard boil eggs, string cheese, yogurt, etc. that needs to be eaten that same day, just stuff it in your lunch bag with the rest of your lunch that day. Eat it if you are hungry and if you don't that day, bring it home and refrigerate it for the next day.

As a reminder, remember to continue all the other rules we have discussed so far.

Rule 9

Rule 9 may be simple for some and hard for others. This rule recommends that you ***avoid eating after 7pm*** to limit additional intake of often empty calories from snacking. I know this may be hard with our busy work schedule during the week, but try your best. The reason for this rule is some of us may tend to continue snacking and eating after dinner. After having a well-balanced dinner with proteins (pork, chicken or fish) with veggies, it should be filling, so that you do not feel hungry to snack. What I often hear from my patients is that they would eat dinner about 8 or 9 o'clock, then go to bed around 10-11pm. Basically, if we eat too late and go to sleep within 1-2 hours, then it often doesn't allow our body enough time to metabolize the food. Because of this, then the food would sit in our stomach undigested and it is harder to burn the calories while sleeping. Also, undigested food sitting in the stomach, especially greasy and fatty meals, will often cause heartburn problems. By avoiding food after 7pm, this will also limit additional consumption of often empty calories/snacking.

If you can't meet the 7pm deadline for dinner, then try to schedule dinner about ½ hour earlier than your usual time. Or after dinner, if you would like a snack, try a frozen yogurt, instead of ice cream or some fruits instead of cookies/chips.

For majority of us, we work an 8am-5pm work schedule, so this is what I am doing. Once I get home around 6pm, I would go straight to preparing dinner. I don't worry about bills or laundry or what happened with the neighbors that day. My focus is to get the meal on the table for dinner before 7pm. During that time, my husband has to take care of the children while I cook. My dishes are very simple and easy to prepare, so we would routinely eat around 6:30 or 6:45pm. Of course, even our best plans do not always go without a hitch, for example, if my child is sick that day or I work late, but majority of the time we are able to make the deadline.

Several tips to be successful with this rule is to try to prep your food the night before (when the kids are asleep) or semi-cook your meals during the weekend and freeze them. See what works best for your schedule. For me, I would do both. I would sometimes marinate my pork/chicken/ fish 1-2 nights in advance or pre-wash and cut my veggies on the weekends when I first buy them (put them in a ziplock bag to keep them as fresh as possible).

As for children, especially for those who regularly snack after dinner, it will be hard the first week with them constantly nagging "why", but just explain to them that it is not healthy. During the second week, it will be easier, like everything else, with practice.

Rule 10

Rule 10 will probably be one of the hardest rule, but very do-able. For Rule 10, I would like you to *cook dinner 1-2 times per week* (Monday-Friday). My definition of "cooking" requires pots/pans and raw meat/veggies. I know I have to specify what cooking means because some people may think getting a frozen burrito or pizza from the freezer and throwing it in the microwave consists of cooking. Again, I'm requesting this rule to be implemented during the weekdays because I would like you to learn to incorporate it in your daily routine. For those you cook every day, this will be easy. But, now focus on incorporating as many fresh ingredients as possible. For those who do not cook on a regular basis, then try to implement this rule during the weekends when you have more time; whatever works for you. Then try to slowly incorporate it into your weekday routine.

The reason I am implementing this plan is because I believe that cooking a simple and healthy meal is a life skill. As you know, the food that is prepared at home tends to be healthier with less fat/salt and we eat in smaller portions. Plus, there is a sense of accomplishment after spending some time cooking and eating the hard work. You know the exact ingredients that are in your food. Of course, practice makes perfect, so don't be discouraged if the meal doesn't turn out right. You can only learn from your mistakes and get better next time. Also, if you have children, when you cook, then they will take an interest in cooking and this will be a great family activity. In addition, as your children gets older and goes off to college, they will be familiar with simple cooking techniques or recipes, so that they won't be dependent on fast food or a microwave to do their "cooking".

Cooking requires planning ahead and this is how I would suggest you to implement the plan. For me, I do my grocery shopping during the weekend. For those who cook on a regular basis, it is easy to go to the store without a shopping list, get what you want, and have complete full meals during the week. But for novices, like me (I'm getting better), I would recommend planning ahead. Write down several ideas or recipes you would like to cook during the week. Have your spouse and children give suggestions what they want to eat as well. Go to the store during the weekend, gather your ingredients and supplies. On Sunday night, try to prepare the ingredients for the week's meals. For the meat/veggies, wash and cut as much as possible. Put it in a container or zip lock bag, then put it back in the refrigerator. Therefore, when you get right home from work on Monday evening, you can just use all the prepared ingredients and cook that night's meal, probably in 1/2 hour. Another option is to use a crock pot. So if you prepare the ingredients on Sunday, then Monday morning before you head off to work, you can toss all the ingredients in the crock pot and have a delicious meal by the time you get home. There are amazing simple recipes online, so experiment.

Basically, the more cooking you do at home, the healthier you will eat! If you are already cooking 1-2 meals/week, then increase it to 2-3 meals/week. I usually only need to cook 3-4 dinners per week and the rest of the days, we are eating leftovers from the previous nights.

For those who do not cook regularly, just try it and you will be amazed. I tell my son that cooking is like magic because from some raw/plain ingredients, you can make yummy food.

Here are some tips for cooking at home:

1. Cook larger portions; eat half of it and freeze the other half for another day. Soups and spaghetti sauce are perfect examples.
2. Share/Rotate cooking duties with your husband and older children; there is no rule that mommies have to do all the cooking

3. Share cleaning duties with your husband and older children; if one cooks, then the other cleans; so cooking doesn't seem like a "chore"
4. Each meal should be simple, but should include a protein (meat/tofu), veggies, and starch (rice, pasta, bread); just remember to limit your amount of starches
   - for example, instead of just eating mac and cheese for dinner, add some strips of chicken breast (you can get it pre-cooked in some warehouse stores) and steam some broccoli/veggies to eat on the side; if you have the protein and veggies, then cut the portion of the mac and cheese.
   - for sphagetti, add steam veggies to the side at meal time or cut mushrooms, onions, bell peppers, zucchini and cook it in the sauce to make it chunkier, so you will use less ground beef. For the ground beef, after browning/cooking it, pour out the excess fat prior to putting the veggies and sauce in.

5. Dinner leftovers make great lunches for the next day (this is what I usually do)
6. Plan, shop, and prepare (as much as you can) during the weekend, so that you just have to cook during the weekday
7. Baking, grilling, stir-frying or pan-searing (frying with a very little amount of oil) is obviously better than anything that is deep fried

Here are some very simple recipes I have gathered from some friends and family that you can try. The main requirements for these recipes are to be as simple as possible and can be prepared in 30minutes. Ask family members or friends to share one quick healthy recipe that they enjoy making for their families. This is a great way to swap your recipes with others, as well.

Jessica's Rotisserie Chicken

1. Buy cooked rotisserie chicken from store
2. Make a salad
3. Cook some frozen veggies

Lisa's Chicken and Couscous

1. Cut chicken breast into slices; cook with very small amount of olive oil
2. Cook instant couscous (Lisa prefers the Israeli type) in fat free chicken broth
3. Cook sliced baby bok choy in a pan with some soy sauce and sesame oil and add pepper
4. At end, stir in a tiny amount of sesame seed

Angelina's Chicken Adobo

1. Cook boneless/skinless chicken in water
2. When chicken is cooked, then shred in small pieces
3. Put chicken in a sauce pan, then add lemon, soy sauce, and seasonings and stir
4. Eat over rice with veggies on side

Angelina's Taco

1. Cook chicken or ground turkey (add little salt/pepper to taste; taco sauce?)
2. Shred cheese; cut tomatoes and lettuce
3. Make your taco with above ingredients
4. Add light sour cream/avocado (optional)

Chrystyne's Salmon and Spinach

1. Season a fillet of salmon (can use any fish you would like or fillet of chicken/pork/turkey) with either just salt and pepper OR with anyone of Ms. Dash's seasoning (let sit for 10-15minutes)
2. Wash fresh spinach; cook spinach with a little bit of olive oil (or canola oil)

3. Cook the salmon/chicken/pork/turkey in a frying pan in a little bit of olive oil (or canola oil)
4. Eat with rice

Chrystyne's StirFry

1. Cut and wash broccoli; small slices of carrots; cut yellow onion
2. Cut slices of beef or chicken; season with little salt and pepper
3. Stir fry (cook) broccoli/carrots/onion together with with soysauce or oyster sauce; take out of pan when done
4. Cook beef or chicken until done, then add the cooked veggies to mix
5. Eat with rice

Nguyet's Chicken with Caesar Orzo and veggies

1. Wash and pat dry two fillets of chicken breasts. Season lightly with salt and pepper. In a skillet, add olive oil and brown both sides of the chicken, should be about 3-4 minutes on each side at medium heat. Remove from skillet and keep warm.
2. In the same skillet, pour in 1 cup of chicken broth; heat to boil. Add in 1/2 cup of Orzo pasta and reduce heat. Stir occasionally for 8-10 minutes. In the meantime, wash and slice baby carrots and asparagus in 1 inch segments. Add in with Orzo. Stir for 1 minute. Add 2 tbs of Caesar dressing and stir. 3. Add chicken back in for another 5 minutes. Stir occasionally or pasta will stick. Remove from heat and serve. This serves for two people.

Tracey's Chinese Chicken Salad (good for parties)

Spring Mix Package
Rotisserie Chicken (Shredded)
Cucumber

Cherry or Grape tomatoes
1 can mandarin orange
chow mein

dressing-
2/3 cup teriyaki sauce (i like kikkoman brand)
2/3 cup white vinegar (i use rice wine vinegar)
1 cup canola oil
6 tablespoon sugar
1/2teapoon salt and 1/2 teaspoon pepper
1/2 cup sesame seeds

LeeAnn's hearty vegetable soup:
1 can of diced tomato with juice
1 box of chicken broth/stock (or 3 cans of broth/stock)
1-2 cups of frozen vegetables from a bag OR any fresh veggies (I used bell peppers onions and broccoli)
1 diced potato
1/2 cup of corn
1 cup of shredded chicken (I used rotisserie) OR raw, cut into small chunks of chicken
3/4 cup of dried pasta (preferably something small like elbow or bow tie)
Salt/pepper to taste

Directions:

1) Pour chicken broth into a soup pot and bring to a boil. Add in diced potato and the veggies. Cook until tender.
2) When the potato is 3/4 done add the pasta. Cook pasta in the broth; this will slightly thicken the soup making for a nice consistency.
3) Add diced tomatoes, corn, and chicken. Simmer. Add salt and pepper to taste.

The journey continues

Even though, my 10 rules have come to an end, this is not definitely the end of your journey. For some, this plan may have taken 5-6months to complete, for others, it may be longer. You may have lost only 10 pounds or 20pounds in total, so far, but again, this is not the end of your journey. My ultimate goal is for you to maintain your current weight loss for a lifetime by continuing the healthy habits that you have established in the 10 rules. For those who want to do more and further advance your weight loss goals, you will need to look at the previous rules and increase the intensity. For example, if you were walking/exercising 30mins/day before, increase to 45mins/day. If you were doing 30mins of walking, you can increase the intensity by adding weights or start jogging or running. Or if you were bringing your lunch only 2-3 x/day, maybe increase it to 4-5x/day. Again, just implement each new change every 2weeks.

You now have momentum on your side and you are smarter about your lifestyle and food choices, so don't give up.

Also, this is a good time to look into other unhealthy habits like smoking or drinking alcohol. Seek your medical professional's help if necessary. There is never a shame in trying to improve yourself.

This plan is designed for adults, but as you can see around you, majority of our children are also overweight and obese. We can only teach by example. From now on, **CHOOSE to EAT LESS and MOVE MORE** and your children will, too.

CHRYSTYNE TRAN, MSPA-C